CONQUERING CANCER:

A COMPREHENSIVE GUIDE TO UNDERSTANDING AND FIGHTING THE DISEASE

DIPAN KUMAR DAS

SUDIP KUMAR DAS

This book is dedicated to all those who have been affected by cancer—patients, survivors, caregivers, families, and friends. It is a tribute to your strength, resilience, and unwavering spirit in the face of adversity.

To the patients, you are the warriors who fight the battle with courage, determination, and grace. Your journey is a testament to the power of the human spirit and the will to live. May your strength inspire others and may you find healing, hope, and comfort along the way.

To the survivors, you are beacons of light and symbols of triumph. Your stories of resilience and perseverance are a source of inspiration for others walking a similar path. May your journey serve as a reminder that there is life beyond cancer and that hope is always within reach.

To the caregivers, you are the unsung heroes providing unwavering love, support, and care. Your selflessness and compassion make a profound difference in the lives of those you care for. May you find strength in knowing the impact you have on the lives of your loved ones and may you find solace in the community of caregivers who understand your journey.

To the families and friends, you provide the unwavering support, love, and encouragement that is essential on the cancer journey. Your presence and understanding offer solace and strength during the most challenging times. May you continue to be pillars of support and sources of comfort for your loved ones.

To the researchers, healthcare professionals, and advocates, your dedication to advancing cancer research, treatment, and support services is changing lives. Your tireless efforts bring hope and promise to those affected by cancer. May you continue to push the boundaries of knowledge, uncover breakthroughs, and shape a future where cancer is conquered.

Finally, this book is dedicated to the memory of those who have lost their lives to cancer. Your legacies live on, and your stories serve as a reminder of the urgent need for continued research, support, and advocacy. May we honor your memory by working tirelessly to create a future where no more lives are lost to this devastating disease.

Together, let us stand united in the fight against cancer, offering support, love, and hope to all those affected. May this dedication serve as a tribute to the resilience, strength, and unity of the cancer community.

Foreword

Preface

Prologue

1.

What Is Cancer?

2.

Understanding Cancer Treatment Options

3.

Early Detection And Prevention Of Cancer

4.

Coping With Cancer Diagnosis And Treatment

5.

Living With Cancer

6.

Innovative Cancer Research And Treatment Breakthroughs

7.

Cancer And Society

8.

Personal Stories Of Surviving Cancer

9.

Cancer And The Future

Epilogue: A Message Of Hope

Foreword

In the face of cancer, words often fall short in capturing the range of emotions, experiences, and challenges that individuals and their loved ones encounter. Cancer is a disease that knows no boundaries, affecting people of all ages, backgrounds, and walks of life. It brings forth fear, uncertainty, and a multitude of questions.

As I reflect upon the pages of this book, I am reminded of the profound impact that cancer has on individuals, families, and society as a whole. It is a journey filled with ups and downs, triumphs and setbacks, hope and despair. Yet, amidst the hardships, there is an undeniable strength that emerges—an indomitable spirit that unites patients, survivors, caregivers, and advocates in a shared mission to overcome this disease.

This book serves as a comprehensive guide, shedding light on the various aspects of cancer. From its causes and risk factors to the latest advancements in research and treatment, it offers a wealth of knowledge and insights. It addresses the physical, emotional, and practical challenges faced by those affected by cancer, while also highlighting the importance of early detection, lifestyle changes, and support systems.

Through its chapters, the book explores the different treatment modalities, ranging from surgery to immunotherapy, and provides guidance on managing the physical symptoms and side effects that may arise. It delves into the emotional impact of cancer, the importance of support for patients and their families, and the strategies for coping with the uncertainty of recurrence.

In addition, the book looks beyond individual experiences and delves into the societal impact of cancer. It touches upon the role of government policies, the need for increased research funding, and the power of advocacy in shaping a future where cancer is preventable, treatable, and ultimately defeated.

Within these pages, you will also find stories of inspiration and resilience—narratives that speak to the triumph of the human spirit in the face of adversity. These stories remind us that while cancer may bring challenges, it also brings forth remarkable strength, courage, and hope. They demonstrate the power of community, compassion, and unwavering support.

As you embark on this journey through the pages of this book, I encourage you to approach it with an open heart and an inquisitive mind. Whether you are a patient seeking knowledge, a caregiver seeking guidance, or simply someone looking to gain a deeper understanding of this disease, may these words provide solace, support, and enlightenment.

Above all, may this book inspire a sense of unity—a reminder that we are all in this fight against cancer together. Let us stand shoulder to shoulder, supporting one another, advocating for change, and fostering a future where cancer no longer casts its dark shadow upon our lives.

In closing, I extend my deepest gratitude to all those who have contributed to this book—the researchers, healthcare professionals, caregivers, survivors, and advocates who have dedicated their lives to the fight against cancer. Your unwavering commitment is a beacon of hope, illuminating the path towards a brighter future.

May this book serve as a source of empowerment, guidance, and inspiration for all who read it. Together, let us forge ahead with determination, compassion, and unwavering hope.

Preface

Cancer. The word alone evokes a range of emotions and experiences, touching the lives of countless individuals around the world. It is a disease that has shaped the lives of patients, survivors, caregivers, families, and communities. It is a disease that calls for understanding, empathy, and action.

In writing this book, our aim is to provide a comprehensive resource that explores the various aspects of cancer—from its causes and risk factors to its prevention, detection, and treatment. We delve into the physical, emotional, and societal impact of cancer, offering insights, guidance, and support for those affected by this disease.

We recognize that every cancer journey is unique, shaped by individual circumstances, medical advancements, and personal choices. Through the chapters in this book, we aim to provide a broad understanding of the multifaceted nature of cancer, while also emphasizing the importance of personalized care and individualized approaches.

Within these pages, you will find information on the different types of cancer, their stages, and the various treatment modalities available. We explore the role of surgery, radiation therapy, chemotherapy, immunotherapy, targeted therapy, and hormone therapy in fighting cancer. We discuss the importance of early detection, the significance of lifestyle changes in reducing cancer risk, and the vital role of support systems for patients and their families.

Throughout the book, we integrate the latest developments in cancer research and treatment, shedding light on promising advancements and breakthroughs that offer hope for a future without cancer. We emphasize the importance of continued research, government policies, and community support in driving progress and improving outcomes for those affected by cancer.

It is important to note that while this book provides valuable information, it does not replace professional medical advice. Each individual's cancer journey is unique, and treatment decisions should be made in consultation with healthcare professionals who can provide personalized guidance based on specific circumstances.

We would like to express our heartfelt gratitude to the researchers, healthcare professionals, caregivers, and cancer survivors who have contributed their expertise and shared their stories throughout the creation of this book. Your insights and experiences have enriched its content and offered valuable perspectives.

Lastly, we dedicate this book to all those who have been affected by cancer—the patients who face this disease with bravery and resilience, the survivors who inspire us with their stories of hope and triumph, the caregivers who provide unwavering support and care, and the families and friends who stand by their side. It is our hope that this book serves as a source of knowledge, support, and encouragement as you navigate the challenges of cancer.

Together, let us strive for a future where cancer is preventable, treatable, and ultimately cured. Let us foster a community of compassion, understanding, and unity. And let us extend our collective hand to those who need it most, offering solace, support, and the promise of a brighter tomorrow.

Prologue

In the vast tapestry of human existence, there are moments that test our resolve, challenge our strength, and push us to the very limits of our being. A cancer diagnosis is one such moment—a seismic shift that disrupts lives, shatters illusions, and propels individuals and their loved ones into a world filled with uncertainty, fear, and resilience.

The journey through cancer is a labyrinth of emotions, marked by highs and lows, triumphs and setbacks, and moments of unimaginable courage. It is a path that demands unwavering strength, unyielding hope, and the unbreakable bonds of support.

In this prologue, we embark upon a voyage—an exploration of the world of cancer. Together, we will navigate the intricacies of its causes, its impact, and the ever-evolving landscape of its prevention, detection, and treatment.

We will meet individuals who have stared into the face of cancer and found the strength to fight back. We will witness their stories of resilience, endurance, and survival—

testaments to the human spirit's indomitable will.

Throughout these pages, we will uncover the latest advancements in research and treatment, shining a light on the groundbreaking discoveries and innovations that hold promise for a future without cancer. We will delve into the depths of scientific inquiry, exploring the intricacies of cancer biology and the intricately woven tapestry of targeted therapies, immunotherapies, and precision medicine.

But this book is more than a compendium of knowledge. It is a testament to the power of community—the compassion and support that unite us in the face of adversity. It is a call to action—a call to rally around those affected by cancer, to lift them up, to provide solace and understanding, and to work tirelessly towards a world where cancer no longer casts its shadow.

As we turn the page and embark upon this journey, let us approach it with open hearts and open minds. Let us be guided by empathy, compassion, and a profound desire for change. And let us be reminded that even in the face of the darkest of storms, there is always a glimmer of hope—a beacon that guides us towards a future where cancer is but a memory.

In the chapters that follow, we invite you to explore, to learn, and to be inspired. Together, let us traverse the vast landscape of cancer, illuminating the way with knowledge, understanding, and unwavering determination.

CHAPTER ONE
What is Cancer?

- Definition of cancer

Cancer can be defined as a complex group of diseases characterized by the uncontrolled growth and spread of abnormal cells in the body. Normally, cells grow and divide in an orderly manner to replace old or damaged cells. However, in the case of cancer, this process goes awry, leading to the formation of a mass of tissue called a tumor.

Tumors can be either benign or malignant. Benign tumors are non-cancerous and typically do not spread to other parts of the body. They can be removed and, in most cases, do not pose a significant threat to health. On the other hand, malignant tumors are cancerous and have the ability to invade nearby tissues and spread to other parts of the body through a process called metastasis.

Cancer can occur in virtually any part of the body and can affect various organs and systems. It is a complex disease with many different types, including breast cancer, lung cancer, prostate cancer, colorectal cancer, and many others. Each type of cancer may have unique characteristics, risk factors, and treatment approaches.

The development of cancer is often influenced by a combination of genetic, environmental, and lifestyle factors. These factors can include genetic mutations, exposure to carcinogens (such as tobacco smoke or certain chemicals), chronic inflammation, certain infections, unhealthy diet, lack of physical activity, and other individual-specific factors.

Early detection and diagnosis of cancer are crucial for successful treatment and improved outcomes. Various screening methods, such as mammography, colonoscopy, and Pap smears, help detect cancer at an early stage when it is more treatable. Treatment options for cancer may include surgery, radiation therapy, chemotherapy, immunotherapy, targeted therapy, and hormone therapy. The choice of treatment depends on the type and stage of cancer, as well as the individual's overall health.

Cancer research continues to advance our understanding of the disease and improve treatment options. Significant progress has been made in recent years, leading to improved survival rates and quality of life for many cancer patients. However, cancer remains a significant health challenge globally, and ongoing efforts are needed to prevent, detect, and treat this complex disease effectively.

- Causes and risk factors

The development of cancer is a complex process influenced by a variety of causes and risk factors. While it is not always possible to identify the exact cause of an individual's cancer, several factors have been associated with an increased risk of developing the disease. Here are some common causes and risk factors of cancer:

1. Genetic Factors: Certain inherited gene mutations can increase the risk of developing specific types of cancer. For example, mutations in the BRCA1 and BRCA2 genes are

associated with a higher risk of breast and ovarian cancer.

2. Age: The risk of developing cancer generally increases with age. This is due to accumulated genetic changes and prolonged exposure to risk factors over time.

3. Environmental and Occupational Exposures: Exposure to certain chemicals, toxins, and substances in the environment or workplace can increase the risk of cancer. Examples include asbestos, benzene, tobacco smoke, radiation, and certain industrial chemicals.

4. Lifestyle Choices:

Tobacco Use: Smoking or using tobacco products is a leading cause of various types of cancer, including lung, mouth, throat, and bladder cancer.

Unhealthy Diet: Poor dietary choices, such as a high intake of processed foods, red and processed meats, sugary beverages, and low intake of fruits and vegetables, are associated with an increased risk of certain cancers.

Lack of Physical Activity: Insufficient physical activity has been linked to a higher risk of several types of cancer, including colorectal, breast, and endometrial cancer.

Alcohol Consumption: Regular and excessive alcohol consumption is a known risk factor for several cancers, including those of the liver, breast, and colon.

5. Chronic Inflammation: Chronic inflammation, which can arise from conditions like chronic infections, autoimmune diseases, or prolonged exposure to irritants, can increase the risk of certain cancers. For instance, chronic hepatitis infections can lead to liver cancer.

6. Hormonal Factors: Hormonal imbalances or prolonged exposure to certain hormones can increase the risk of specific cancers. For example, long-term use of hormone replacement therapy (HRT) in menopause has been associated with an increased risk of breast and ovarian cancer.

7. Family History: A family history of certain types of cancer, particularly in first-degree relatives (parents, siblings, children), can indicate a genetic predisposition and an increased risk of developing cancer.

It's important to note that having one or more of these risk factors does not necessarily mean that an individual will develop cancer. Many individuals without identifiable risk factors still develop cancer, while others with several risk factors never do. However, understanding these causes and risk factors can help individuals make informed decisions about their lifestyle choices, undergo appropriate screening tests, and engage in early detection and preventive measures to reduce their risk of developing cancer.

- Different types of cancer

There are numerous types of cancer, each originating in specific cells or tissues within the body. Here is an overview of some common types of cancer:

1. Breast Cancer: Breast cancer forms in the cells of the breast and is predominantly found in women. It can also occur in men, albeit less frequently. Breast cancer may present as a lump or thickening in the breast tissue and can spread to nearby lymph nodes.

2. Lung Cancer: Lung cancer develops in the tissues of the lungs, typically due to long-term exposure to tobacco smoke, but it can also occur in non-smokers. There are two primary types: non-small cell lung cancer (NSCLC) and small cell lung cancer (SCLC). Lung cancer is a leading cause of cancer-related deaths worldwide.

3. Prostate Cancer: Prostate cancer originates in the prostate gland, which is part of the male reproductive system. It is one of the most common cancers in men. Prostate cancer often grows slowly and may not cause symptoms initially, but it can be aggressive in some cases.

4. Colorectal Cancer: Colorectal cancer affects the colon or rectum and usually begins as a polyp, a noncancerous growth. Over time, these polyps can become cancerous. Colorectal cancer can cause changes in bowel habits, rectal bleeding, abdominal pain, and unexplained weight loss.

5. Melanoma: Melanoma is a type of skin cancer that develops in melanocytes, the pigment-producing cells of the skin. It often starts as a mole or dark spot that undergoes changes in shape, color, or size. Melanoma can spread rapidly to other parts of the body if not detected and treated early.

6. Leukemia: Leukemia is a cancer of the blood and bone marrow, characterized by the abnormal production of white blood cells. It affects the body's ability to produce healthy blood cells, leading to symptoms such as fatigue, frequent infections, easy bleeding, and anemia.

7. Lymphoma: Lymphoma is a cancer that originates in the lymphatic system, which is responsible for fighting infections. There are two main types of lymphoma: Hodgkin lymphoma and non-Hodgkin lymphoma. Lymphomas typically present as swollen lymph nodes, unexplained weight loss, fever, and night sweats.

8. Pancreatic Cancer: Pancreatic cancer begins in the pancreas, an organ involved in digestion and hormone regulation. It is often diagnosed at an advanced stage, making it challenging to treat. Common symptoms include abdominal pain, weight loss, jaundice, and digestive problems.

9. Ovarian Cancer: Ovarian cancer arises in the ovaries, which are part of the female reproductive system. It may cause symptoms such as abdominal bloating, pelvic pain, frequent urination, and changes in menstrual cycles. Ovarian cancer is often diagnosed at an advanced stage.

10. Bladder Cancer: Bladder cancer affects the bladder, the organ

responsible for storing urine. It commonly presents with symptoms like blood in the urine, frequent urination, pain during urination, and lower back pain.

These are just a few examples of the many types of cancer that can affect different organs and systems in the body. Each type of cancer has its own unique characteristics, risk factors, diagnostic methods, and treatment approaches. It is essential to consult with healthcare professionals for accurate diagnosis, treatment planning, and personalized care.

- Stages of cancer

Cancer staging is a system used to describe the extent and spread of cancer within the body. It helps determine the severity of the disease, guide treatment decisions, and provide prognostic information. The most commonly used cancer staging system is the TNM system, which stands for Tumor, Node, and Metastasis. Here's an overview of the stages in cancer:

Stage 0: This stage, also known as carcinoma in situ, refers to abnormal cells that are present only in the layer of cells where they first developed and have not invaded nearby tissues. Stage 0 cancers are considered non-invasive.

Stage I: At this stage, cancer is usually small in size and localized to the organ where it originated. It has not spread to nearby lymph nodes or distant sites. Stage I cancers are often highly treatable.

Stage II: Cancer at this stage is larger in size or has invaded nearby tissues but has not spread to the lymph nodes or distant sites. The extent of local invasion determines the subcategories of Stage II.

Stage III: In Stage III, cancer has typically spread to nearby lymph nodes but not to distant sites. The extent of lymph node involvement and local invasion determines the subcategories of Stage III.

Stage IV: Stage IV indicates that cancer has spread to distant organs or distant lymph nodes. It is considered advanced or metastatic cancer. Stage IV is further divided into subcategories based on the specific locations and extent of metastasis.

Apart from the TNM system, some cancers have their own staging systems based on specific characteristics and considerations. For example, staging systems for hematological cancers like leukemia and lymphoma may involve factors such as cell type, genetic abnormalities, and specific markers.

It's important to note that the staging system can vary for different types of cancer. Some cancers may have additional staging criteria, while others may have simplified staging systems. The specific staging information for a particular type of cancer can be obtained from medical professionals who specialize in the disease.

Cancer staging plays a crucial role in determining treatment options, predicting prognosis, and assessing the effectiveness of therapies. It helps healthcare providers tailor treatment plans to individual patients and monitor the progression or regression of the disease over time.

CHAPTER TWO
Understanding Cancer Treatment Options

- Surgery

Surgery is a primary treatment modality for cancer and is often used to remove tumors and surrounding tissues. It plays a crucial role in the diagnosis, staging, and treatment of various types of cancer. The specific surgical approach depends on factors such as the type, location, and stage of cancer, as well as the overall health of the patient. Here are some important aspects of cancer surgery:

Diagnostic Surgery: In some cases, surgery is performed to obtain a sample of tissue for diagnosis. This is known as a biopsy, and it helps determine if a tumor is cancerous and provides information about its type and characteristics.

Curative Surgery: Curative surgery aims to completely remove the tumor and any affected surrounding tissues. This is often performed when cancer is localized and has not spread to distant sites. The goal is to eliminate the cancer and achieve long-term remission or cure.

Debulking Surgery: In cases where complete removal of the tumor is not possible, debulking surgery is performed to remove as much of the tumor as feasible. This can help reduce the size of the tumor, alleviate symptoms, and improve the effectiveness of other treatments like chemotherapy or radiation therapy.

Palliative Surgery: Palliative surgery is performed to relieve symptoms and improve the quality of life for patients with advanced cancer. It may involve removing a portion of the tumor or addressing complications caused by the cancer, such as pain, obstruction, or bleeding.

Lymph Node Surgery: Cancer often spreads to nearby lymph nodes, so surgical removal and examination of lymph nodes may be necessary to determine the extent of cancer and guide further treatment decisions. This procedure is called lymphadenectomy or lymph node dissection.

Reconstructive Surgery: In cases where surgical removal of a tumor results in significant cosmetic or functional deficits, reconstructive surgery may be performed to restore the appearance or function of the affected area. This can involve techniques such as tissue grafting, reconstruction with implants, or plastic surgery procedures.

Minimally Invasive Surgery: Minimally invasive techniques, such as laparoscopic or robotic-assisted surgery, are increasingly used in cancer treatment. These procedures involve smaller incisions, specialized instruments, and cameras for visualization, resulting in reduced scarring, shorter recovery times, and less post-operative pain.

Surgery is often combined with other treatments like radiation therapy, chemotherapy, immunotherapy, or targeted therapy, depending on the type and stage of cancer. It is essential to discuss the benefits, risks, and potential outcomes of surgery with a surgical oncologist or a multidisciplinary team of healthcare professionals to determine the most appropriate treatment approach for each individual case.

- Radiation therapy

Radiation therapy, also known as radiotherapy, is a cancer treatment that uses high-energy radiation to kill or damage cancer cells. It is a localized treatment method that targets the tumor site while minimizing damage to surrounding healthy tissues. Radiation therapy can be used at different stages of cancer treatment and in various forms. Here are some key points about radiation therapy:

External Beam Radiation Therapy: This is the most common form of radiation therapy. It involves the use of a machine called a linear accelerator to deliver radiation from outside the body. The machine directs high-energy X-rays or other types of radiation precisely to the tumor site. Treatment sessions are typically scheduled over several weeks, with each session lasting only a few minutes.

Internal Radiation Therapy (Brachytherapy): In internal radiation therapy, radioactive materials are placed directly into or near the tumor site. This can be done using implants, capsules, or radioactive seeds. The radiation emitted from these sources delivers a higher dose of radiation to the tumor while reducing exposure to surrounding healthy tissues. Brachytherapy may be temporary (the sources are removed after a specific time) or permanent (the sources remain in the body).

Intensity-Modulated Radiation Therapy (IMRT): IMRT is an advanced technique that delivers radiation with varying intensities, allowing for precise targeting of the tumor while minimizing exposure to nearby healthy tissues. It uses computer-controlled devices to shape the radiation beams and deliver them from multiple angles.

Stereotactic Radiosurgery (SRS) and Stereotactic Body Radiation Therapy

(SBRT): These are highly precise radiation therapy techniques used to treat small tumors with a high dose of radiation in a single or few sessions. SRS is typically used for brain tumors, while SBRT is used for tumors in other parts of the body.

Adjuvant Radiation Therapy: Adjuvant radiation therapy is given after surgery to eliminate any remaining cancer cells and reduce the risk of recurrence. It is commonly used in breast, lung, and colorectal cancers, among others.

Neoadjuvant Radiation Therapy: Neoadjuvant radiation therapy is administered before surgery to shrink tumors and make them more amenable to surgical removal. It can be used in various types of cancer, such as rectal cancer or locally advanced breast cancer.

Palliative Radiation Therapy: Palliative radiation therapy aims to relieve symptoms and improve the quality of life for patients with advanced cancer. It is often used to alleviate pain, reduce tumor size, control bleeding, or alleviate other cancer-related symptoms.

Radiation therapy may have side effects, which vary depending on the area being treated and the dose of radiation. Common side effects can include fatigue, skin changes, hair loss (in the treated area), nausea, and temporary or long-term effects on organ function. The treatment team will work closely with the patient to manage side effects and provide supportive care.

Radiation therapy is typically planned and administered by a radiation oncologist in collaboration with a multidisciplinary team of healthcare professionals. The decision to use radiation therapy, its timing, and the specific technique employed depend on the type, stage, and location of cancer, as well as the patient's overall health. The treatment plan is tailored to each individual to optimize outcomes and minimize side effects.

- Chemotherapy

Chemotherapy is a systemic cancer treatment that uses drugs to kill cancer cells or stop them from growing and dividing. Unlike surgery or radiation therapy, which target specific areas, chemotherapy circulates throughout the body and can reach cancer cells that have spread to distant sites. Here are some key points about chemotherapy:

How It Works: Chemotherapy drugs work by interfering with the cell division process, either by damaging the DNA or disrupting other essential cellular processes. By targeting rapidly dividing cells, chemotherapy aims to destroy cancer cells while also affecting normal cells that divide quickly, such as those in the bone marrow, hair follicles, and the lining of the gastrointestinal tract.

Administration: Chemotherapy can be given in different ways, depending on the type of cancer and the specific drugs used. It may be administered orally in the form of pills or capsules, through injections into a vein (intravenous), through injections into a muscle (intramuscular), or as topical creams or gels. The treatment schedule can vary, with cycles of chemotherapy followed by rest periods to allow the body to recover.

Combination Therapy: In many cases, chemotherapy drugs are used in combination to increase effectiveness and reduce the likelihood of drug resistance.

Different drugs with varying mechanisms of action may be combined to target cancer cells at various stages of the cell cycle or to attack cancer cells in different ways.

Adjuvant and Neoadjuvant Chemotherapy: Adjuvant chemotherapy is given after surgery or other primary treatments to kill any remaining cancer cells and reduce the risk of recurrence. Neoadjuvant chemotherapy, on the other hand, is given before surgery to shrink tumors and facilitate surgical removal.

Systemic Effects: Chemotherapy drugs can have side effects due to their impact on normal cells. Common side effects include fatigue, nausea and vomiting, hair loss, decreased blood cell counts (resulting in increased risk of infection, anemia, or bleeding), and gastrointestinal issues. However, advances in supportive care have helped to manage these side effects better, and not all patients experience the same level of side effects.

Targeted Therapies: In recent years, targeted therapies have emerged as a subset of chemotherapy. These drugs specifically target cancer cells by blocking specific molecules or pathways involved in cancer growth and progression. Targeted therapies are designed to be more selective and less toxic to normal cells, potentially resulting in fewer side effects.

Chemotherapy is used in the treatment of various types of cancer, including but not limited to breast cancer, lung cancer, colorectal cancer, leukemia, lymphoma, and ovarian cancer. The specific chemotherapy drugs and regimen are determined based on the type and stage of cancer, overall health of the patient, and individualized treatment plans.

It's important to note that chemotherapy is a rapidly evolving field, and new drugs and treatment approaches continue to be developed. The treatment team, including oncologists and oncology nurses, closely monitors patients during chemotherapy, adjusts the treatment as needed, and provides supportive care to manage side effects and optimize treatment outcomes.

- Immunotherapy

Immunotherapy is an innovative cancer treatment approach that utilizes the body's immune system to recognize, target, and destroy cancer cells. Unlike traditional cancer treatments that directly target cancer cells, immunotherapy enhances the immune response to effectively combat cancer. Here are some key points about immunotherapy:

Principles of Immunotherapy: The immune system has the ability to recognize abnormal cells, including cancer cells, and mount an immune response against them. However, cancer cells can develop mechanisms to evade the immune system. Immunotherapy works by stimulating or restoring the immune system's ability to recognize and attack cancer cells.

Checkpoint Inhibitors: One of the main types of immunotherapy is checkpoint inhibitors. Normally, there are proteins on immune cells called checkpoints that regulate immune responses and prevent excessive immune reactions. However, cancer cells can exploit these checkpoints to evade immune detection. Checkpoint inhibitors block these proteins, such as PD-1 (programmed cell death protein 1) or

CTLA-4 (cytotoxic T-lymphocyte-associated protein 4), allowing immune cells to recognize and attack cancer cells more effectively.

CAR-T Cell Therapy: CAR-T (chimeric antigen receptor T-cell) therapy is a form of immunotherapy that involves modifying a patient's own T cells to express a specific receptor on their surface. This receptor allows the T cells to recognize and target cancer cells with a specific antigen. CAR-T cell therapy has shown promising results in the treatment of certain blood cancers, such as leukemia and lymphoma.

Cancer Vaccines: Cancer vaccines are another type of immunotherapy that aim to stimulate the immune system to recognize and attack cancer cells. These vaccines can be composed of cancer cell components, antigens, or immune-stimulating substances. They can help train the immune system to specifically target cancer cells and initiate an immune response against them.

Adoptive Cell Transfer: Adoptive cell transfer involves collecting and modifying a patient's immune cells, such as T cells, in the laboratory and then reintroducing them into the patient's body. These modified immune cells are engineered to better recognize and destroy cancer cells. This approach has shown promising results in the treatment of certain cancers, such as melanoma.

Immune Checkpoint Modulators: In addition to checkpoint inhibitors, other immune checkpoint modulators are being developed and studied. These include agents that target different immune checkpoints or molecules involved in immune regulation. These modulators aim to enhance the immune response against cancer cells and improve treatment outcomes.

Indications and Side Effects: Immunotherapy has been approved for the treatment of various cancers, including melanoma, lung cancer, kidney cancer, bladder cancer, and more. However, not all patients or cancer types respond equally to immunotherapy. Side effects of immunotherapy can occur and vary depending on the specific treatment used and individual patient factors. Common side effects include fatigue, rash, flu-like symptoms, and inflammation of organs, among others. However, serious side effects are less common.

Combination Approaches: Immunotherapy is often used in combination with other treatments, such as chemotherapy, targeted therapy, or radiation therapy, to enhance treatment effectiveness. Combining different treatment modalities can lead to synergistic effects and improve overall treatment outcomes.

Immunotherapy is a rapidly evolving field, and ongoing research continues to explore new approaches and combinations to optimize its effectiveness. The decision to use immunotherapy is based on several factors, including the type and stage of cancer, the patient's overall health, and biomarkers or characteristics of the tumor. The treatment plan is personalized to each patient's specific needs and may involve a multidisciplinary team of healthcare professionals, including medical oncologists and immunologists.

- Targeted therapy

Targeted therapy is a form of cancer treatment that specifically targets the unique characteristics or vulnerabilities of cancer cells while minimizing damage to normal cells. Unlike chemotherapy, which affects rapidly dividing cells in general, targeted therapy focuses on the specific molecules or pathways that play a critical role in cancer growth and progression. Here are some key points about targeted therapy:

Molecular Targets: Targeted therapy drugs are designed to interact with specific molecules or proteins that are present in cancer cells or their surrounding environment. These targets can include receptor proteins on the surface of cancer cells, intracellular signaling pathways, or specific genetic mutations or abnormalities.

Types of Targeted Therapy: There are different types of targeted therapy approaches, including:

1. Small Molecule Inhibitors: These drugs are typically taken orally and can enter cells to block specific signaling pathways or target molecules inside the cells.

2. Monoclonal Antibodies: These drugs are designed to bind to specific targets on cancer cells, either directly killing the cells or signaling the immune system to destroy them.

3. Signal Transduction Inhibitors: These drugs interfere with the

signaling pathways that promote cancer cell growth and survival.

4. Angiogenesis Inhibitors: These drugs target the formation of new blood vessels that supply nutrients and oxygen to tumors, thereby inhibiting their growth.

5. PARP Inhibitors: These drugs target a specific DNA repair enzyme called poly ADP-ribose polymerase (PARP) and are effective in cancers with specific DNA repair defects.

Patient Selection: Targeted therapies are often guided by specific biomarkers or genetic mutations found in the tumor. Before starting targeted therapy, patients may undergo genetic testing or other molecular profiling to identify the presence of actionable targets that can be effectively targeted by available drugs.

Combination Approaches: Targeted therapies can be used alone or in combination with other treatments, such as chemotherapy, radiation therapy, or immunotherapy. Combinations of targeted therapies may also be used to address multiple molecular targets simultaneously or to overcome potential resistance mechanisms.

Effectiveness and Side Effects: Targeted therapies have shown significant efficacy in certain cancers, particularly those with well-defined molecular targets. They can lead to improved treatment outcomes, including tumor shrinkage, prolonged survival, and better quality of life. However, as with any treatment, targeted therapies can have side effects, which vary depending on the specific drugs used and the individual patient. Common side effects may include skin reactions, gastrointestinal issues, hypertension, or other specific side effects related to the targeted pathway or molecule.

Ongoing Research and Personalized Medicine: The field of targeted therapy is rapidly evolving, and ongoing research aims to identify new targets and develop more effective drugs. The goal is to move toward a personalized medicine approach where treatment decisions are based on the specific molecular characteristics of each patient's tumor.

It is important to consult with an oncologist or a healthcare professional specializing in targeted therapy to determine the suitability of targeted therapy for an individual's specific cancer type and circumstances. The treatment plan will be personalized based on the patient's molecular profile, tumor characteristics, and other relevant factors.

- Hormone therapy

Hormone therapy, also known as endocrine therapy, is a cancer treatment approach that uses medications to block or interfere with the hormones that fuel the growth and spread of certain types of cancer. It is primarily used in the treatment of hormone receptor-positive cancers, such as breast cancer and prostate cancer, where hormones like estrogen or testosterone play a significant role in tumor development and progression. Here are some key points about hormone therapy:

Hormone Receptor-Positive Cancers: Certain cancers, such as breast cancer and prostate cancer, have receptors on their cells that can bind to hormones like estrogen or testosterone. These hormones stimulate the growth of cancer cells. Hormone receptor-positive cancers express these hormone receptors, making them susceptible to hormone therapy.

Goals of Hormone Therapy: The primary goals of hormone therapy are to slow down or stop the growth of hormone receptor-positive cancer cells, reduce the risk of recurrence, and manage cancer symptoms. In some cases, hormone therapy may be used as a neoadjuvant treatment before surgery to shrink tumors or as an adjuvant treatment after surgery to reduce the risk of cancer recurrence.

Types of Hormone Therapy:

1. Anti-Estrogen Therapy: Anti-estrogen therapy is commonly used in the treatment of hormone receptor-positive breast cancer. Drugs like tamoxifen and aromatase inhibitors (such as letrozole, anastrozole, or exemestane) block the estrogen receptors or reduce estrogen production, thus depriving the cancer cells of estrogen stimulation.

2. Anti-Androgen Therapy: Anti-androgen therapy is used in the treatment of prostate cancer. Drugs like bicalutamide, flutamide, or enzalutamide block the binding of testosterone or other androgens to the androgen receptors in prostate cancer cells, thereby slowing down tumor growth.

3. Luteinizing Hormone-Releasing Hormone (LHRH) Agonists or Antagonists: These medications are used in prostate cancer to lower testosterone levels. LHRH agonists, such as leuprolide or goserelin, initially cause an increase in hormone levels followed by a decrease, while LHRH antagonists like degarelix directly lower hormone levels.

Duration of Treatment: Hormone therapy may be given for a specific duration, such as a few years, or it may be continued indefinitely, depending on the cancer type, stage, and other individual factors. Treatment duration and decisions regarding when to stop or switch therapies are based on ongoing assessments and discussions with the healthcare team.

Side Effects: Hormone therapy can have side effects, which vary depending on the specific medications used and the individual patient. Common side effects may include hot flashes, night sweats, sexual dysfunction, fatigue, bone thinning (osteoporosis), mood changes, weight gain, or joint pain. It's important to communicate any side effects to the healthcare team to manage them effectively.

Combination Therapies: Hormone therapy is sometimes combined with other treatments, such as surgery, radiation therapy, or chemotherapy, depending on the specific cancer type, stage, and treatment plan. Combination therapies can enhance treatment effectiveness and outcomes.

Monitoring and Follow-up: Regular monitoring and follow-up visits are important during hormone therapy to assess treatment response, manage side effects, and make any necessary adjustments to the treatment plan. This ensures optimal treatment outcomes and patient well-being.

It's important to consult with an oncologist or a healthcare professional specializing in hormone therapy to determine the most appropriate treatment approach for an individual's specific cancer type and situation. The treatment plan will be personalized based on the tumor characteristics, hormone receptor status, patient preferences, and other relevant factors.

CHAPTER THREE

Early Detection and Prevention of Cancer

- Importance of early detection

Early detection plays a crucial role in the management and treatment of cancer. Detecting cancer at an early stage offers several important benefits:

1. Increased Treatment Options: Early detection often allows for a wider range of treatment options. When cancer is diagnosed at an early stage, it is generally localized and more likely to be treatable with curative intent. Treatment options may include less aggressive therapies, such as localized surgery or radiation therapy, which can help preserve organ function and improve overall quality of life.

2. Improved Treatment Outcomes: Early detection is associated with

better treatment outcomes. By detecting cancer in its early stages, there is a higher chance of complete removal or destruction of the cancerous cells, leading to higher cure rates and increased survival rates. Early treatment can prevent the cancer from spreading to other parts of the body (metastasis), which is typically associated with poorer prognoses.

3. Reduced Treatment Intensity: Early detection may reduce the need for extensive treatment interventions. In some cases, early-stage cancers may require less aggressive treatments, such as smaller surgical procedures or lower doses of radiation or chemotherapy. This can

minimize the physical and emotional impact of treatment, reduce potential side effects, and improve overall patient well-being.

4. Cost Savings: Early detection can lead to cost savings in cancer care. Early-stage cancers are generally less complex to treat, requiring fewer medical resources and interventions. This can result in lower healthcare costs for patients, healthcare systems, and insurance providers.

5. Increased Long-Term Survival: Early detection is often associated with improved long-term survival rates. When cancer is diagnosed early and treated effectively, the chances of long-term remission and survival

are significantly higher. Regular cancer screenings and awareness of potential signs and symptoms can contribute to earlier detection, leading to better long-term outcomes.

6. Psychological and Emotional Benefits: Early detection can provide peace of mind and reduce anxiety. Timely diagnosis allows patients to proactively address their condition, seek appropriate medical support, and engage in informed decision-making regarding their treatment. It can also provide an opportunity for emotional and psychological support, as patients can access counseling or join support groups early in their cancer journey.

To promote early detection, it is important to raise awareness about the signs and symptoms of various cancers, encourage regular screenings, and provide accessible healthcare services for early detection and diagnosis. Regular check-ups, screenings, and following recommended guidelines for cancer screenings based on age, gender, and risk factors are essential for early detection and improved outcomes.

• Screening tests for common types of cancer

Screening tests are used to detect cancer in individuals who do not have any symptoms. These tests aim to identify cancer at an early stage when treatment is often more effective. Here are some common screening tests for specific types of cancer:

1. Breast Cancer:

Mammography: A mammogram is an X-ray of the breast tissue used to detect breast cancer. It is recommended for women starting at the age of 40 or earlier for those with higher risk factors.

Clinical Breast Examination (CBE): A healthcare provider examines the breasts for any abnormalities or lumps during a physical examination.

2. Cervical Cancer:

Pap Smear (Pap Test): This test involves collecting cells from the cervix to check for abnormalities or pre-cancerous changes. It is typically recommended for women starting at the age of 21 and repeated at regular intervals as advised by healthcare providers.

3. Colorectal Cancer:

Colonoscopy: This procedure uses a flexible tube with a camera to examine the entire colon and rectum for polyps or signs of cancer. It is generally recommended starting at the age of 50, with follow-up intervals based on the findings.

Fecal Occult Blood Test (FOBT): This test checks for hidden blood in the stool, which can be an early sign of colorectal cancer. It is recommended annually or as advised by healthcare providers.

4. Lung Cancer:

Low-Dose Computed Tomography (LDCT): This imaging test uses low-dose X-rays to create detailed images of the lungs and is recommended for individuals at high risk for lung cancer, typically aged 55 to 80 with a history of smoking.

5. Prostate Cancer:

Prostate-Specific Antigen (PSA) Test: This blood test measures the level of PSA, a protein produced by the prostate gland. It is used to detect abnormalities in the prostate, including prostate cancer. The decision to undergo PSA testing is typically based on shared decision-making between the individual and their healthcare provider.

It's important to note that the recommendations for screening tests may vary depending on factors such as age, gender, family history, and individual risk factors. It is advisable to consult with healthcare professionals or primary care physicians who can provide personalized guidance on the appropriate screening tests and schedules based on an individual's specific circumstances.

• Lifestyle changes to reduce the risk of cancer

Making certain lifestyle changes can help reduce the risk of developing cancer. While it's important to note that no lifestyle modification can guarantee the prevention of cancer, adopting healthy habits can contribute to overall well-being and lower the risk of cancer. Here are some lifestyle changes that can help reduce the risk:

1. Avoid Tobacco: Tobacco use is a leading cause of many types of cancer, including lung, mouth, throat, esophageal, and pancreatic cancer. Quitting smoking and avoiding secondhand smoke are crucial steps in reducing cancer risk. Seek support from healthcare professionals or

support groups to aid in smoking cessation.

2. Maintain a Healthy Weight: Obesity and excess body weight have been linked to an increased risk of several types of cancer, including breast, colorectal, ovarian, and pancreatic cancer. Maintaining a healthy weight through regular physical activity and a balanced diet can help reduce the risk. Aim for a body mass index (BMI) within the healthy range.

3. Eat a Healthy Diet: A well-balanced diet rich in fruits, vegetables, whole grains, and lean proteins can help lower the risk of certain cancers. Include a variety of colorful fruits and vegetables in your

meals, limit processed and red meats, choose whole grains over refined grains, and reduce consumption of sugary beverages and processed foods.

4. Engage in Regular Physical Activity: Regular physical activity has been associated with a reduced risk of several types of cancer, including breast, colon, and lung cancer. Strive for at least 150 minutes of moderate-intensity aerobic activity or 75 minutes of vigorous-intensity aerobic activity per week. Incorporate strength training exercises twice a week.

5. Protect Yourself from the Sun: Exposure to ultraviolet (UV) radiation from the sun increases the

risk of skin cancer, including melanoma. Protect your skin by seeking shade, wearing protective clothing, using sunscreen with a high SPF, and avoiding indoor tanning beds.

6. Limit Alcohol Consumption: Alcohol consumption is linked to an increased risk of several types of cancer, including breast, liver, and colorectal cancer. If you choose to drink alcohol, do so in moderation. The American Cancer Society recommends limiting alcohol to no more than one drink per day for women and two drinks per day for men.

7. Practice Safe Sex and Get Vaccinated: Certain sexually

transmitted infections, such as human papillomavirus (HPV) and hepatitis B, are associated with an increased risk of developing certain cancers. Practice safe sex, get vaccinated against HPV, and follow recommended vaccination schedules for hepatitis B to reduce the risk.

8. Get Regular Screenings: Following recommended cancer screening guidelines is vital for early detection and treatment. Regular screenings can detect cancer at an early stage or even precancerous conditions, improving the chances of successful treatment. Consult with healthcare professionals to determine the appropriate screenings based on

age, gender, and individual risk factors.

Remember, incorporating these lifestyle changes into your daily routine can have a positive impact on your overall health and well-being, reducing the risk of cancer and improving overall quality of life.

• Vaccines for cancer prevention

Vaccines play a crucial role in cancer prevention by protecting against certain viral infections that are known to cause or contribute to the development of certain types of cancer. Here are some vaccines that can help prevent cancer:

1. Human Papillomavirus (HPV) Vaccine: HPV is a sexually

transmitted infection that can cause various cancers, including cervical, vaginal, vulvar, penile, anal, and some types of throat and mouth cancers. The HPV vaccine protects against the most common types of HPV that cause cancer. It is recommended for both males and females in their early teenage years, ideally before they become sexually active. Catch-up vaccinations may be recommended for older individuals who have not yet received the vaccine.

2. Hepatitis B Vaccine: Chronic infection with the hepatitis B virus (HBV) can lead to liver damage and an increased risk of liver cancer. The hepatitis B vaccine is highly effective

in preventing HBV infection. It is recommended for all infants at birth and for individuals who may be at increased risk of exposure to the virus, such as healthcare workers, individuals with multiple sexual partners, and those who inject drugs.

3. Other Vaccines: Although not primarily designed for cancer prevention, certain vaccines indirectly reduce the risk of cancer by preventing infections associated with cancer development. For example:

• The measles, mumps, and rubella (MMR) vaccine helps prevent measles, which in rare cases can lead to a type of cancer called measles inclusion-body encephalitis-associated lymphoma.

- The varicella (chickenpox) vaccine prevents chickenpox and its complications, including the rare occurrence of cancer, such as lymphoma or skin cancer, in individuals with weakened immune systems.

It's important to note that vaccines provide the best protection when administered before exposure to the respective viruses. Vaccination programs and schedules may vary by country, and it's recommended to consult with healthcare professionals or follow national immunization guidelines to determine the appropriate vaccines and schedules based on age, gender, and individual risk factors.

In addition to vaccines, it's important to maintain regular screenings, follow healthy lifestyle practices, and practice safe behaviors to further reduce the risk of cancer. Vaccines, along with other preventive measures, contribute to the overall efforts in reducing the burden of cancer in populations.

CHAPTER FOUR

Coping with Cancer Diagnosis and Treatment

- Emotional impact of cancer

The emotional impact of cancer can be profound and far-reaching, affecting not only the individuals diagnosed with cancer but also their loved ones and caregivers. Coping with a cancer diagnosis and undergoing treatment can evoke a range of emotions that may vary throughout the cancer journey. Here are some common emotional experiences and challenges associated with cancer:

1. Fear and Anxiety: The diagnosis of cancer often triggers fear and anxiety about the future, treatment outcomes, and the potential impact on one's life. Uncertainty about the disease and its progression can contribute to heightened anxiety levels.

2. Depression and Sadness: Cancer can lead to feelings of sadness, hopelessness, and depression. Coping with the physical symptoms, treatment side effects, and the disruption of daily life can contribute to emotional distress.

3. Grief and Loss: Cancer may involve a sense of loss, including the loss of good health, independence, body image, and roles within relationships or work. Grieving these losses is a natural response to the challenges posed by cancer.

4. Stress and Overwhelm: Cancer can be an overwhelming experience, with numerous medical appointments, treatment decisions, and financial burdens. Coping with

these stressors can be challenging and may lead to feelings of being overwhelmed.

5. Anger and Frustration: Cancer diagnosis can evoke feelings of anger and frustration, directed towards the disease itself, treatment difficulties, or even towards loved ones or healthcare providers. These emotions may arise from a sense of injustice or the disruption of life plans.

6. Body Image and Self-esteem: Cancer treatments, such as surgery, radiation, or chemotherapy, can cause physical changes that impact body image and self-esteem. Coping with these changes and adjusting to a new self-image can be emotionally challenging.

7. Social Isolation and Loneliness: Cancer may lead to social isolation as individuals navigate treatment schedules, side effects, and physical limitations. Fear of judgment or the inability to participate in previous social activities can contribute to feelings of loneliness.

8. Post-Traumatic Stress: Some individuals may experience post-traumatic stress symptoms after a cancer diagnosis, particularly if they have had a traumatic experience related to their diagnosis, treatment, or medical procedures.

It's important to recognize and address these emotional challenges. Seeking emotional support from healthcare professionals, counselors, support groups, or loved ones can be beneficial. These resources can provide a safe space to express emotions, offer coping strategies, and provide guidance for managing the emotional impact of cancer. Additionally, self-care practices such as relaxation techniques, exercise, maintaining social connections, and engaging in activities that bring joy and a sense of purpose can help individuals navigate the emotional journey of cancer.

• Dealing with the physical symptoms and side effects of treatment

Dealing with the physical symptoms and side effects of cancer treatment is an important aspect of the cancer journey. While the specific symptoms and side effects can vary depending on the type of cancer and treatment received, here are some general strategies for managing them:

1. Communicate with Your Healthcare Team: Open and honest communication with your healthcare team is essential. They can provide information about potential side effects, offer strategies for managing them, and adjust treatment plans if necessary. Be sure to report any symptoms or side effects promptly so that they can be addressed.

2. Follow Medication and Treatment Guidelines: Take medications as prescribed and follow the recommended treatment

schedule. This can help manage side effects and optimize the effectiveness of the treatment.

3. Manage Pain: If you experience pain, discuss it with your healthcare team. They can prescribe appropriate pain medications or recommend alternative pain management strategies, such as physical therapy, acupuncture, or relaxation techniques.

4. Eat a Healthy Diet: Proper nutrition is crucial during cancer treatment. A balanced diet with a variety of nutrient-rich foods can help support your immune system, maintain energy levels, and promote healing. If you have specific dietary concerns or side effects that affect

eating, such as nausea or loss of appetite, consult with a registered dietitian for personalized guidance.

5. Stay Hydrated: Drinking enough fluids is important, especially if you are experiencing side effects such as vomiting or diarrhea. Stay hydrated by sipping water throughout the day and considering hydrating beverages or electrolyte-replenishing solutions if recommended by your healthcare team.

6. Manage Nausea and Vomiting: If you experience nausea and vomiting, your healthcare team can prescribe anti-nausea medications or suggest other strategies like eating smaller, more frequent meals, avoiding strong

smells, and trying relaxation techniques.

7. Fatigue Management: Cancer treatments can often cause fatigue. Prioritize rest and sleep, and try to balance activity with periods of rest. Engage in gentle exercise, such as walking or yoga, if approved by your healthcare team, as it can help combat fatigue.

8. Emotional Support: Physical symptoms and side effects can take a toll on your emotional well-being. Seek emotional support from loved ones, support groups, or mental health professionals who can help you navigate the challenges and provide coping strategies.

9. Maintain Personal Hygiene: Good personal hygiene practices, such as regular bathing, oral care, and skincare, can help prevent infections and improve overall well-being during treatment.

10. Follow Guidelines for Activity and Exercise: Depending on your condition and treatment, your healthcare team may provide guidelines for physical activity and exercise. Follow their recommendations to maintain strength, manage side effects, and improve overall physical and mental well-being.

Remember, everyone's experience with treatment side effects is unique. It's important to work closely with your healthcare team to address and manage your specific symptoms and side effects effectively. They can provide personalized guidance and support throughout your cancer treatment journey.

• Support for cancer patients and their families

Support for cancer patients and their families is crucial in helping them navigate the challenges and emotional impact of the disease. Here are some avenues of support that can be beneficial:

1. Healthcare Team: The primary healthcare team, including doctors, nurses, and other healthcare professionals, play a vital role in

providing medical care, treatment information, and support. They can address concerns, provide guidance on treatment options, and help manage side effects.

2. Supportive Care Services: Many healthcare facilities have supportive care services or departments dedicated to addressing the holistic needs of cancer patients and their families. These services may include palliative care, pain management, psychosocial support, counseling, and complementary therapies like massage, acupuncture, or art therapy.

3. Support Groups: Joining cancer-specific support groups or community-based organizations allows individuals and their families

to connect with others who are going through similar experiences. Sharing experiences, emotions, and coping strategies in a supportive environment can be empowering and comforting.

4. Counseling and Mental Health Support: Professional counseling services, such as psychologists or social workers, can provide emotional support and help individuals and families navigate the complex emotions and challenges associated with cancer. They offer coping strategies, address concerns, and provide a safe space to express fears, grief, or anxiety.

5. Online Communities: Online platforms and forums provide a

virtual space for individuals and families affected by cancer to connect, share experiences, and offer support. These communities can be valuable for seeking information, finding resources, and building relationships with others facing similar challenges.

6. Patient Navigators: Patient navigators or oncology nurses can assist individuals and families in understanding treatment plans, scheduling appointments, coordinating care, and accessing support services. They serve as a point of contact and help navigate the healthcare system.

7. Financial Assistance: Cancer treatment can impose significant

financial burdens. There are organizations and resources available that provide financial assistance or guidance on managing the costs associated with treatment, such as insurance, medication, transportation, and other related expenses.

8. Faith-Based Support: Religious or spiritual communities can offer comfort, prayer support, and counseling services to individuals and families dealing with cancer. Seek support from clergy members or faith-based organizations that provide spiritual guidance and assistance.

9. Friends and Family: The support of loved ones is invaluable. Family and friends can provide emotional

support, assist with practical needs, accompany individuals to medical appointments, and offer a listening ear during difficult times.

10. Respite and Caregiver Support: Caring for a loved one with cancer can be physically and emotionally demanding. Caregiver support programs and respite care services can provide relief, guidance, and resources for caregivers to take care of their own well-being.

It's important for individuals and families to proactively seek and utilize the available support services. Different people find different types of support helpful, so it's essential to find what works best for your specific needs and preferences.

Remember, you don't have to face cancer alone, and reaching out for support is a sign of strength.

CHAPTER FIVE

Living with Cancer

- Managing life after diagnosis and treatment

Managing life after a cancer diagnosis and treatment can present unique challenges as individuals transition into a new phase of survivorship. Here are some important aspects to consider when navigating life after cancer:

1. Follow-Up Care: Regular follow-up appointments with your healthcare team are essential to monitor your health, detect any potential recurrence or new health concerns,

and address any lingering side effects of treatment. Follow the recommended surveillance and screening guidelines specific to your cancer type.

2. Emotional Well-being: The emotional impact of cancer can continue even after treatment ends. Seek emotional support through counseling, support groups, or individual therapy to address any lingering emotional challenges, anxiety, depression, or fear of recurrence. Focus on self-care practices, stress management techniques, and engage in activities that promote well-being and positive mental health.

3. **Physical Fitness and Healthy Lifestyle:** Maintain a healthy lifestyle to optimize overall well-being. Engage in regular physical activity, as recommended by your healthcare team, to improve strength, endurance, and overall fitness. Adopt a balanced diet with emphasis on whole foods, fruits, vegetables, and lean proteins. Limit alcohol consumption, avoid tobacco use, and protect yourself from excessive sun exposure.

4. **Fatigue Management:** Cancer-related fatigue can persist even after treatment. Prioritize rest, listen to your body's needs, and establish a healthy sleep routine. Plan activities and conserve energy by pacing

yourself throughout the day. Engage in gentle exercises, such as walking or yoga, to improve energy levels and combat fatigue.

5. Body Image and Self-Esteem: Adjusting to physical changes that may have occurred during treatment can be challenging. Seek support from healthcare professionals, support groups, or therapists who can provide guidance on coping with body image concerns and rebuilding self-esteem.

6. Career and Employment: Returning to work or making career adjustments after cancer treatment may require careful consideration. Communicate with your employer about any necessary workplace

accommodations or modifications. Consider seeking vocational counseling or career guidance to explore potential career transitions or adjustments that align with your post-treatment needs and goals.

7. Relationships and Support: Nurture relationships with family, friends, and support networks. Openly communicate with loved ones about your experiences, needs, and concerns. Join cancer survivorship programs, connect with other survivors, and engage in support groups to find a sense of community and shared experiences.

8. Financial and Insurance Matters: Evaluate your financial situation and consider seeking assistance if

needed. Discuss insurance coverage, medical bills, and financial planning with financial advisors, social workers, or patient advocacy organizations to ensure you have the necessary support and resources.

9. Set Goals and Celebrate Milestones: Set realistic goals and celebrate milestones in your cancer journey. Whether it's returning to a favorite hobby, planning a trip, or pursuing new interests, having goals and celebrating achievements can provide a sense of purpose and optimism for the future.

10. Survivorship Care Plan: Work with your healthcare team to develop a survivorship care plan that outlines the specific follow-up care,

screenings, and lifestyle recommendations tailored to your individual needs and cancer history. This plan serves as a roadmap for managing your ongoing healthcare and addressing any potential long-term effects of cancer treatment.

Remember, the transition to life after cancer is a unique and personal journey. Be patient with yourself, seek support when needed, and embrace the opportunities for growth, resilience, and a renewed appreciation for life.

- Coping with cancer recurrence

Coping with cancer recurrence can be a challenging and emotional experience. Here are some strategies to help you navigate this difficult time:

1. Acknowledge and Express Your Emotions: Allow yourself to experience and acknowledge the range of emotions that may arise, including fear, anger, sadness, and anxiety. It's normal to feel a mix of emotions when facing a recurrence. Find healthy outlets to express your emotions, such as talking to a trusted friend or family member, joining a support group, or seeking professional counseling.

2. Seek Information: Learn as much as you can about the recurrence, including the available treatment options and their potential outcomes. Consult with your healthcare team to

understand the specifics of your situation, ask questions, and discuss your concerns. Knowledge can help alleviate some of the uncertainties and empower you to make informed decisions.

3. Establish a Support System: Lean on your support system, including friends, family, and healthcare professionals. Share your feelings and concerns with them and allow them to provide comfort and support. Consider joining support groups or online communities where you can connect with others who have experienced cancer recurrence. They can offer empathy, understanding, and practical advice based on their own experiences.

4. Communicate with Your Healthcare Team: Maintain open and honest communication with your healthcare team. Share any new symptoms or concerns promptly and ask for clarification or additional information about your treatment options. Engage in shared decision-making with your doctors to ensure your treatment plan aligns with your goals and preferences.

5. Take Care of Your Physical and Emotional Well-being: Prioritize self-care during this time. Focus on healthy habits, including regular exercise, balanced nutrition, sufficient sleep, and stress management techniques such as meditation or deep breathing

exercises. Engage in activities that bring you joy, relaxation, and a sense of normalcy.

6. Set Realistic Expectations: Understand that coping with cancer recurrence is a process that takes time. Be patient with yourself and set realistic expectations. It's normal to have good and bad days emotionally. Allow yourself to grieve, but also find moments of hope and positivity.

7. Explore Complementary Therapies: Complementary therapies like acupuncture, massage, yoga, or mindfulness practices may help reduce stress, alleviate physical symptoms, and improve overall well-being. Discuss these options with your healthcare team to determine

their appropriateness and potential benefits for your specific situation.

8. Embrace Supportive Services: Utilize supportive care services, such as palliative care, pain management, or counseling services, to address any physical, emotional, or spiritual needs that arise. These services can help improve your quality of life, manage symptoms, and provide holistic support.

9. Find Meaning and Support in Survivorship: Embrace the concept of survivorship and find meaning in your journey. Engage in activities or projects that bring a sense of purpose, whether it's advocacy work, supporting others going through similar experiences, or pursuing

personal goals and passions. Celebrate each day and find joy in the present moment.

10. Practice Self-Compassion: Be kind to yourself throughout the recurrence journey. Recognize that you are doing the best you can in a difficult situation. Treat yourself with compassion and allow yourself the space to heal emotionally and physically.

Remember, coping with cancer recurrence is highly individual, and everyone's experience is unique. Find what strategies work best for you and seek the support and resources that can help you navigate this challenging time.

- Tips for a healthy lifestyle during and after treatment

Maintaining a healthy lifestyle during and after cancer treatment is essential for overall well-being and recovery. Here are some tips to support a healthy lifestyle:

1. Balanced Diet: Aim for a balanced diet that includes a variety of fruits, vegetables, whole grains, lean proteins, and healthy fats. Focus on nutrient-dense foods to support your immune system and aid in the healing process. Limit processed foods, sugary snacks, and saturated fats.

2. Hydration: Drink an adequate amount of water throughout the day

to stay hydrated. Proper hydration supports various bodily functions, helps manage side effects like constipation, and promotes overall well-being.

3. Regular Exercise: Engage in regular physical activity as recommended by your healthcare team. Exercise can help improve strength, manage fatigue, reduce stress, and enhance overall quality of life. Choose activities that you enjoy, such as walking, swimming, yoga, or cycling, and gradually increase intensity and duration based on your comfort level.

4. Rest and Sleep: Prioritize rest and aim for quality sleep. Adequate rest and sleep are essential for

healing and recovery. Establish a relaxing bedtime routine, create a comfortable sleep environment, and seek support if you are experiencing sleep difficulties.

5. Stress Management: Find effective ways to manage stress during and after treatment. Engage in stress-reducing activities such as meditation, deep breathing exercises, yoga, or engaging in hobbies that bring joy and relaxation. Consider techniques like mindfulness or guided imagery to promote mental and emotional well-being.

6. Tobacco and Alcohol: Avoid tobacco use and limit or avoid alcohol consumption. Both tobacco and excessive alcohol intake can

have detrimental effects on your health and increase the risk of cancer recurrence and other health complications.

7. Sun Protection: Protect your skin from the harmful effects of the sun by wearing protective clothing, applying sunscreen with a high SPF, and seeking shade during peak sun hours. This helps reduce the risk of skin cancer and protects sensitive skin during and after treatment.

8. Regular Check-ups: Attend follow-up appointments and screenings as recommended by your healthcare team. Regular check-ups help monitor your health, detect any potential issues early, and ensure timely intervention if needed.

9. Emotional Well-being: Prioritize your emotional well-being by seeking support, whether through counseling, support groups, or connecting with loved ones. Engage in activities that promote relaxation, self-care, and self-expression to help manage stress and improve overall mental health.

10. Gradual Lifestyle Changes: Make changes to your lifestyle gradually and sustainably. Set realistic goals and focus on making long-term, positive changes rather than adopting extreme or restrictive measures. Seek guidance from healthcare professionals, including registered dietitians or exercise

specialists, for personalized advice and support.

Remember, everyone's journey is unique, and it's important to listen to your body and consult with your healthcare team to develop a plan that suits your specific needs and circumstances. Your healthcare team can provide personalized recommendations based on your treatment history, overall health, and individual goals.

CHAPTER SIX

Innovative Cancer Research and Treatment Breakthroughs

- Latest developments in cancer research and treatment

1. Precision Medicine: Precision medicine focuses on tailoring

treatment to an individual's specific cancer characteristics, such as genetic mutations or biomarkers. This approach aims to improve treatment outcomes and reduce side effects by targeting therapies to the unique genetic profile of a patient's tumor.

2. Immunotherapy Advancements: Immunotherapy has shown promising results in treating various types of cancer by boosting the body's immune system to target and destroy cancer cells. Researchers continue to explore new immunotherapeutic approaches, combination therapies, and the identification of novel immune targets.

3. CAR-T Cell Therapy: Chimeric Antigen Receptor T-cell (CAR-T) therapy is a type of immunotherapy that involves modifying a patient's own immune cells to recognize and attack cancer cells. CAR-T therapies have shown significant success in certain types of blood cancers and are being investigated for their potential in other cancer types.

4. Liquid Biopsies: Liquid biopsies involve analyzing a patient's blood sample for circulating tumor cells, circulating tumor DNA, or other biomarkers. This non-invasive approach has the potential to monitor treatment response, detect minimal residual disease, and identify genomic changes in real-time,

allowing for more personalized treatment decisions.

5. Targeted Therapies: Targeted therapies focus on specific molecular alterations in cancer cells that drive tumor growth. Advancements in understanding genetic mutations and signaling pathways have led to the development of targeted therapies that can disrupt these specific pathways, resulting in improved outcomes for certain cancer types.

6. Genomic Profiling: Genomic profiling allows for a comprehensive analysis of a patient's tumor DNA to identify specific genetic alterations. This information can guide treatment decisions and help identify targeted

therapies or clinical trial opportunities.

7. Combination Therapies: Researchers are investigating the effectiveness of combining different treatment modalities, such as chemotherapy, immunotherapy, targeted therapies, and radiation therapy, to enhance treatment response and overcome resistance mechanisms.

8. Novel Drug Development: Pharmaceutical companies and researchers are continuously developing and testing new drugs, including small molecules and biologics, to target different aspects of cancer biology. These include inhibitors of specific signaling

pathways, cancer metabolism, and epigenetic modifications.

9. Artificial Intelligence and Machine Learning: Artificial intelligence and machine learning technologies are being applied to cancer research and treatment to analyze complex data, identify patterns, predict treatment response, and assist in diagnosis and treatment planning.

10. Supportive Care Advances: Efforts are being made to improve supportive care measures to manage the physical and emotional side effects of cancer treatment. This includes advances in pain management, symptom control,

palliative care, and psychosocial support.

It's important to note that ongoing research and advancements in cancer treatment are continually evolving. For the most up-to-date information, I recommend consulting reputable sources such as medical journals, cancer research organizations, and healthcare professionals specialized in oncology.

• Future directions in cancer treatment

1. Immunotherapy Advancements: Immunotherapy has revolutionized cancer treatment, and further advancements are expected. Researchers are exploring

combination immunotherapies, developing more precise immune checkpoint inhibitors, and improving personalized cancer vaccines.

2. Cellular Therapies: Cellular therapies, such as CAR-T cell therapy, are showing promising results in blood cancers. Future directions may include developing off-the-shelf CAR-T products, expanding the use of cellular therapies to solid tumors, and improving safety profiles and long-term outcomes.

3. Targeted Therapies and Precision Medicine: As our understanding of cancer genetics improves, targeted therapies will continue to play a significant role. Future developments

may involve identifying new targets, developing more effective inhibitors, and integrating precision medicine into routine clinical practice.

4. Epigenetic Modifications: Epigenetic alterations play a crucial role in cancer development and progression. Researchers are exploring epigenetic therapies to modify gene expression patterns in cancer cells, potentially leading to new treatment approaches.

5. Liquid Biopsies and Early Detection: Liquid biopsies have the potential to revolutionize cancer detection and monitoring. Future developments may include improving the sensitivity and specificity of liquid biopsy tests,

detecting cancer at earlier stages, and monitoring treatment response and minimal residual disease.

6. Combination Therapies: Combination therapies that target multiple pathways or utilize different treatment modalities (e.g., chemotherapy, targeted therapy, immunotherapy) are being investigated to overcome resistance and improve treatment outcomes. Identifying optimal combinations and understanding their synergistic effects will be a focus of future research.

7. Novel Drug Delivery Systems: Researchers are exploring innovative drug delivery systems to enhance treatment efficacy while minimizing

side effects. This includes nanoparticles, drug-eluting implants, and targeted delivery approaches to improve tumor specificity and reduce toxicity.

8. Artificial Intelligence and Data Analytics: The integration of artificial intelligence (AI) and machine learning in cancer research and treatment is expected to grow. AI can help analyze vast amounts of data, identify patterns, predict treatment outcomes, and assist in clinical decision-making and personalized treatment approaches.

9. Cancer Prevention and Early Intervention: Efforts will continue to focus on cancer prevention strategies, such as lifestyle modifications,

screening programs, and vaccination against cancer-associated viruses. Additionally, early intervention and detection of precancerous lesions or early-stage cancers may lead to more effective and less invasive treatment options.

10. Patient-Centric Approaches: Future cancer treatments will likely emphasize personalized medicine, taking into account individual patient characteristics, preferences, and treatment goals. This includes incorporating patient-reported outcomes, shared decision-making, and supportive care measures to enhance quality of life during and after treatment.

CHAPTER SEVEN
Cancer and Society

- Impact of cancer on society

Cancer has a significant impact on society in various ways. Here are some key aspects:

1. Health and Healthcare Systems: Cancer places a considerable burden on healthcare systems worldwide. The diagnosis, treatment, and management of cancer require substantial resources, including medical personnel, specialized facilities, medications, and supportive care services. The increasing prevalence of cancer and

the complexity of treatments contribute to rising healthcare costs and challenges in providing accessible and equitable cancer care.

2. Economic Impact: Cancer has substantial economic implications for individuals, families, and society as a whole. The direct costs of cancer treatment, including medical expenses and medications, can be substantial. Indirect costs, such as loss of productivity, missed workdays, and caregiver burden, also contribute to the economic impact. Additionally, cancer research and development of new treatments require significant financial investments.

3. Emotional and Psychological Impact: Cancer diagnosis and treatment can have profound emotional and psychological effects on individuals and their families. The experience of cancer often brings feelings of fear, anxiety, depression, grief, and stress. Emotional support, counseling, and mental health services are essential to help individuals and families cope with the emotional impact of cancer.

4. Caregiver Burden: Cancer affects not only individuals with the disease but also their caregivers. Providing care for a loved one with cancer can be physically, emotionally, and financially demanding. Caregivers may experience increased stress,

fatigue, and disruption of their own lives and routines. Supportive services and caregiver resources are crucial to address their needs and mitigate caregiver burden.

5. Productivity and Workforce Impact: Cancer can have a significant impact on an individual's ability to work and their productivity. Treatment regimens may require time off work for medical appointments, surgeries, and recovery periods. Fatigue, side effects of treatment, and long-term effects can affect an individual's capacity to perform their job effectively. Employers and workplaces play a vital role in supporting employees affected by cancer through workplace

accommodations and supportive policies.

6. Research and Innovation: Cancer research drives scientific advancements and innovation in treatment approaches. It requires collaboration between researchers, healthcare providers, pharmaceutical companies, and funding agencies. Societal support and investments in cancer research are crucial to further understanding the disease, developing effective treatments, and improving patient outcomes.

7. Advocacy and Awareness: The impact of cancer on society has led to increased advocacy efforts and public awareness campaigns. These initiatives aim to educate the public

about cancer prevention, early detection, treatment options, and the importance of supportive care. They also advocate for policy changes, funding for research, and access to quality cancer care for all individuals.

8. Survivorship and Quality of Life: With advancements in cancer treatment, more individuals are surviving and living with cancer as a chronic condition. Survivorship programs and support services are essential to address the long-term physical, emotional, and psychosocial needs of cancer survivors. Enhancing the quality of life for cancer survivors is a critical

aspect of cancer care and requires ongoing support and resources.

Cancer's impact on society is complex and multifaceted. Addressing the challenges and improving outcomes for individuals affected by cancer requires a comprehensive approach that involves healthcare systems, policy changes, research advancements, supportive care services, and community engagement.

• Government policies on cancer research and treatment

Government policies play a crucial role in supporting and advancing cancer research and treatment. Here are some key areas where government policies have an impact:

1. Funding for Research: Governments allocate funding for cancer research through various channels, including national research agencies, institutes, and grant programs. Adequate and sustained funding enables scientists and researchers to conduct studies, investigate new treatment approaches, explore prevention strategies, and improve our understanding of cancer biology.

2. Regulation and Drug Approval: Governments establish regulatory bodies to evaluate and approve new cancer drugs and therapies. These agencies ensure that treatments meet

safety and efficacy standards before they can be made available to patients. Rigorous evaluation processes, such as clinical trials, are necessary to assess the benefits and risks of new treatments.

3. Access to Affordable Care: Government policies aim to ensure that individuals have access to affordable and equitable cancer care. This includes measures such as universal healthcare systems, insurance coverage for cancer treatments, and regulations to prevent discrimination based on pre-existing conditions. Government initiatives may also include programs to support low-income individuals, improve

access to screenings, and reduce financial barriers to treatment.

4. Prevention and Awareness Campaigns: Governments invest in public health initiatives to raise awareness about cancer prevention strategies, early detection, and screening programs. These campaigns educate the public about risk factors, encourage healthy lifestyle choices, promote cancer screenings, and disseminate information on available resources and support services.

5. Supportive Care and Survivorship: Government policies can prioritize the provision of supportive care services for cancer patients and survivors. These

services include psychosocial support, palliative care, pain management, and rehabilitation. Policies may also focus on survivorship programs to address the long-term physical, emotional, and social needs of cancer survivors.

6. Data Sharing and Collaboration: Governments can facilitate data sharing and collaboration among researchers, healthcare institutions, and organizations involved in cancer research and treatment. By encouraging the sharing of data and resources, governments foster collaborative research efforts, accelerate scientific discoveries, and promote the development of more

effective treatments and personalized approaches.

7. Tobacco Control and Public Health Initiatives: Governments often implement policies to control tobacco use, a leading cause of cancer. These policies may include restrictions on smoking in public places, tobacco advertising regulations, increased taxes on tobacco products, and public education campaigns to raise awareness about the dangers of smoking.

8. International Collaboration: Governments engage in international collaborations to share knowledge, resources, and best practices in cancer research and treatment. These

collaborations promote the exchange of scientific expertise, facilitate clinical trials, and support efforts to tackle global cancer challenges.

It's important to note that government policies may vary between countries and regions. Different governments have different approaches to cancer research, treatment, and healthcare systems. Policies are shaped by factors such as available resources, healthcare priorities, political considerations, and societal needs. The ultimate goal of government policies in cancer research and treatment is to improve patient outcomes, reduce the burden of cancer, and enhance the overall well-being of individuals and communities affected by the disease.

• Support for cancer patients and their families

Support for cancer patients and their families is crucial to help them navigate the challenges and complexities that come with a cancer diagnosis. Here are some key areas of support:

1. Medical Support: Medical support encompasses a range of services provided by healthcare professionals, including oncologists, nurses, and other specialized practitioners. This support includes cancer diagnosis, treatment planning, and ongoing medical care. It also

involves addressing the physical symptoms and side effects of treatment, pain management, and monitoring treatment response.

2. Emotional Support: Emotional support is essential for cancer patients and their families to cope with the emotional impact of the disease. This support can come from mental health professionals, counselors, support groups, or peer-to-peer networks. Emotional support aims to address anxiety, depression, fear, grief, and other psychological challenges that may arise during the cancer journey.

3. Supportive Care Services: Supportive care services focus on improving the overall well-being and

quality of life of cancer patients. These services may include palliative care, pain management, symptom control, nutritional counseling, rehabilitation, and complementary therapies. Supportive care aims to manage physical and emotional symptoms, enhance comfort, and address the holistic needs of patients.

4. Caregiver Support: Caregivers play a vital role in supporting cancer patients, and they also require assistance and resources to cope with the challenges they face. Caregiver support services may include education, respite care, counseling, and support groups specifically designed to address the needs and concerns of caregivers.

5. Financial Assistance: Cancer treatment can be costly, and financial support is essential to alleviate the financial burden for patients and their families. Government programs, charitable organizations, and foundations may offer financial assistance or resources to help cover medical expenses, prescription costs, and other related costs such as transportation and accommodation during treatment.

6. Practical Support: Practical support involves assisting patients and their families with the logistical aspects of managing cancer. This may include help with navigating healthcare systems, accessing resources and information,

coordinating appointments, and providing transportation assistance.

7. Community and Peer Support: Engaging with other cancer patients and survivors through support groups or online communities can provide a sense of belonging, understanding, and encouragement. Peer support networks allow individuals to share experiences, exchange advice, and find emotional support from those who have gone through similar challenges.

8. Educational Resources: Access to accurate and reliable information is crucial for patients and families to make informed decisions about their cancer journey. Educational resources may include brochures,

websites, online forums, and educational sessions that provide information about cancer types, treatments, side effects, survivorship, and available support services.

9. Advocacy and Navigation: Cancer advocacy organizations and patient navigators can help patients and families navigate the healthcare system, access appropriate resources, and advocate for their needs and rights. They can provide guidance on insurance coverage, treatment options, and help in overcoming barriers to care.

10. End-of-Life Support: For individuals in advanced stages of cancer, end-of-life support and palliative care services are crucial.

These services aim to provide comfort, dignity, and support for patients and their families during the end-of-life stage, including pain and symptom management, emotional support, and assistance with advance care planning.

It's important to note that the availability and scope of support services may vary depending on the healthcare system, geographical location, and individual circumstances. Patients and families should reach out to healthcare providers, cancer support organizations, and community resources to access the support services available to them.

CHAPTER EIGHT

Personal Stories of Surviving Cancer

- Inspirational stories of cancer survivors

Inspirational stories of cancer survivors can provide hope, encouragement, and motivation to others facing similar challenges. Here are a few examples of remarkable cancer survivor stories:

1. Lance Armstrong: Former professional cyclist Lance Armstrong was diagnosed with testicular cancer that had spread to his lungs and brain. Despite the grim prognosis, he underwent rigorous treatment, including surgery and chemotherapy. Armstrong not only survived but

went on to win the Tour de France seven consecutive times, becoming an inspiration for many cancer patients and survivors worldwide.

2. Fran Drescher: Actress Fran Drescher, known for her role in the TV series "The Nanny," was diagnosed with uterine cancer in 2000. After undergoing surgery and chemotherapy, Drescher became an advocate for cancer awareness and early detection. She founded the Cancer Schmancer Movement, an organization focused on prevention, early diagnosis, and policy changes to improve cancer care.

3. Michael C. Hall: Actor Michael C. Hall, best known for his roles in the TV series "Dexter" and "Six Feet

Under," was diagnosed with Hodgkin's lymphoma in 2010. Hall underwent successful treatment and continued his acting career while raising awareness about the disease. His story emphasizes the importance of early detection and the ability to overcome cancer while pursuing one's passions.

4. Scott Hamilton: Olympic figure skater Scott Hamilton was diagnosed with testicular cancer in 1997 and later faced two brain tumors. Despite the challenges, Hamilton remained resilient, underwent surgeries and treatments, and went on to establish the Scott Hamilton CARES Foundation to support cancer research and survivorship programs.

5. Robin Roberts: Television anchor Robin Roberts, co-host of "Good Morning America," was diagnosed with breast cancer in 2007 and later developed a rare blood disorder called myelodysplastic syndrome (MDS). She underwent treatments, including a bone marrow transplant, and publicly shared her journey, inspiring many with her strength and resilience.

6. Melissa Etheridge: Grammy-winning singer-songwriter Melissa Etheridge was diagnosed with breast cancer in 2004. She underwent surgery and chemotherapy while continuing her music career. Etheridge has been vocal about her experience and became an advocate

for breast cancer awareness, emphasizing the importance of early detection and staying positive during treatment.

7. Mark Herzlich: Former professional football player Mark Herzlich was diagnosed with a rare form of bone cancer called Ewing's sarcoma during his college years. After intense treatment, including surgery and chemotherapy, he made a remarkable recovery and went on to play in the NFL for the New York Giants. Herzlich's story showcases determination and resilience in the face of adversity.

These are just a few examples of the many inspirational stories of cancer survivors who have faced and overcome the disease. Each individual's journey is unique, but their stories serve as a reminder that cancer can be overcome, and life can be embraced even after a diagnosis. These stories offer hope, strength, and inspiration to others navigating their own cancer journeys.

• Lessons learned from their journeys

The journeys of cancer survivors offer valuable lessons that can inspire and empower others. Here are some lessons learned from their experiences:

1. Resilience and Determination: Cancer survivors demonstrate immense resilience and

determination in the face of adversity. They face challenging treatments, physical and emotional struggles, and uncertainty about the future. Their journeys teach us the importance of staying strong, never giving up, and finding the inner strength to face challenges head-on.

2. Importance of a Positive Attitude: Many cancer survivors emphasize the power of maintaining a positive attitude throughout their journey. A positive mindset can help individuals cope with the physical and emotional toll of cancer, find hope in difficult times, and stay motivated to overcome obstacles. It is a reminder that optimism and a fighting spirit can make a significant

difference in one's cancer experience.

3. Advocacy and Awareness: Several cancer survivors become advocates, using their experiences to raise awareness, promote early detection, and support others facing cancer. They use their platforms to educate others about the disease, encourage screenings, and push for policy changes to improve cancer care. Their journeys teach us the importance of giving back and making a difference in the lives of others.

4. Importance of Support Systems: Cancer survivors often highlight the critical role of support systems, including family, friends, healthcare

professionals, and support groups. These networks provide emotional support, practical assistance, and a sense of belonging during challenging times. Their stories remind us of the power of community, love, and support in navigating the cancer journey.

5. Mind-Body Connection: Many cancer survivors emphasize the importance of holistic well-being, recognizing the mind-body connection in their healing process. They often incorporate practices such as exercise, meditation, nutrition, and complementary therapies to support their physical and emotional well-being. Their experiences highlight

the significance of taking care of the whole self and prioritizing self-care.

6. Gratitude and Perspective: Cancer survivors often express gratitude for life and a renewed perspective on what truly matters. Their experiences teach us to appreciate the present moment, cherish relationships, and find joy in the small things. They remind us of the resilience of the human spirit and the capacity to find beauty and purpose even in the midst of adversity.

7. Never Underestimate Your Strength: Cancer survivors demonstrate incredible strength and resilience that they may not have known existed within themselves.

Their journeys teach us not to underestimate our own strength and potential. They inspire us to believe in our ability to overcome challenges, adapt to new circumstances, and live life to the fullest.

The lessons learned from the journeys of cancer survivors remind us of the human spirit's remarkable resilience, the power of a positive mindset, the importance of support systems, and the ability to find meaning and purpose in the face of adversity. These lessons can inspire and empower individuals facing their own cancer journeys, offering hope, guidance, and encouragement along the way.

CHAPTER NINE
Cancer and the Future

•   Advances in cancer prevention, detection, and treatment

Advances in cancer prevention, detection, and treatment have significantly improved outcomes for patients and transformed the landscape of cancer care. Here are some notable advances in these areas:

Prevention:

a. Vaccines: Vaccines have been developed to prevent certain types of cancers. For example, the human papillomavirus (HPV) vaccine can prevent HPV infections that lead to cervical, anal, and other cancers. Hepatitis B vaccination also reduces the risk of liver cancer.

b. Lifestyle Modifications: Increasing awareness of cancer risk factors has led to efforts in promoting healthy lifestyles. Public health campaigns encourage smoking cessation, healthy eating habits, regular physical activity, and sun protection, reducing the risk of several types of cancer.

Detection:

a. Screening Tests: Advances in screening tests have enabled the early detection of cancers, improving treatment outcomes. Mammography, Pap smears, colonoscopies, and low-dose computed tomography (LDCT) scans for lung cancer are examples of screening tests that help identify cancers at an earlier, more treatable stage.

b. Liquid Biopsies: Liquid biopsies are minimally invasive tests that detect cancer-related genetic mutations and biomarkers in blood samples. These tests are being developed to aid in early cancer detection, monitor treatment response, and detect cancer recurrence.

Treatment:

a. Targeted Therapies: Targeted therapies are designed to specifically target cancer cells by interfering with specific molecules involved in cancer growth and progression. These therapies have shown remarkable success in treating various cancers, such as breast cancer, lung cancer, and melanoma, improving treatment effectiveness and reducing side effects.

b. Immunotherapy: Immunotherapy harnesses the body's immune system to fight cancer. This approach stimulates the immune response, enhances immune cell activity, or uses engineered immune cells to target cancer cells. Immunotherapies, such as immune checkpoint inhibitors and CAR-T cell therapy, have shown significant success in treating several cancers, including melanoma, lung cancer, and hematological malignancies.

c. Precision Medicine: Precision medicine tailors treatment approaches based on an individual's genetic profile, tumor characteristics, and other factors. Advances in genomic sequencing technologies have enabled the identification of specific mutations or alterations driving cancer growth. This knowledge helps guide treatment decisions, allowing for personalized therapies and improving treatment outcomes.

d. Minimally Invasive and Robotic Surgery: Minimally invasive surgical techniques, such as laparoscopy and robotic surgery, have revolutionized cancer surgery. These approaches offer smaller incisions, reduced blood loss, shorter hospital stays, and faster recovery times compared to traditional open surgeries.

e. Advances in Radiation Therapy: Radiation therapy techniques have evolved to deliver more precise and targeted radiation doses to cancer cells while minimizing damage to healthy tissues. Techniques such as intensity-modulated radiation therapy

(IMRT), stereotactic body radiation therapy (SBRT), and proton therapy allow for greater treatment accuracy and reduced side effects.

f. Novel Drug Development: Pharmaceutical research continues to identify and develop new cancer drugs with improved efficacy and reduced toxicity. The discovery of novel drug targets and the development of combination therapies are expanding treatment options and improving outcomes for many cancer types.

These advances in cancer prevention, detection, and treatment have significantly impacted patient care and survival rates. However, it's important to note that progress varies across cancer types, and there is still much to learn and achieve. Ongoing research and collaboration among scientists, clinicians, and patients are essential to further advance the field and continue improving cancer outcomes.

• Hope for a future without cancer

The vision of a future without cancer is a shared goal that inspires scientists, healthcare professionals, patients, and society as a whole. While eliminating cancer entirely may be a complex challenge, significant progress has been made, and there are reasons for hope:

1. Advances in Research: The field of cancer research is rapidly

evolving, with ongoing breakthroughs in understanding the biology of cancer cells, the tumor microenvironment, and the complex interactions that drive cancer development and progression. This knowledge provides the foundation for developing innovative strategies to prevent, detect, and treat cancer more effectively.

2. Personalized Medicine: The emergence of precision medicine and genomics has paved the way for tailored treatments based on an individual's unique genetic makeup and tumor characteristics. With advancements in genomic sequencing, biomarker identification, and targeted therapies, personalized

treatment approaches are becoming more accessible and effective, leading to improved outcomes for patients.

3. Immunotherapy Breakthroughs: Immunotherapy has revolutionized cancer treatment by harnessing the body's immune system to recognize and attack cancer cells. Recent breakthroughs in immune checkpoint inhibitors, CAR-T cell therapy, and other immunotherapies have shown remarkable success in treating various types of cancers, including previously challenging and aggressive forms.

4. Early Detection Technologies: Early detection plays a crucial role in improving cancer outcomes. Early detection plays a crucial role in improving cancer outcomes.

Innovative technologies such as liquid biopsies, advanced imaging techniques, and molecular diagnostics are continually being developed to detect cancer at its earliest stages when it is more treatable. These advancements hold promise for more effective screening programs and early intervention strategies.

5. Collaborative Efforts: The fight against cancer requires multidisciplinary collaboration among researchers, clinicians, patient advocates, and policymakers. Global initiatives, research networks, and public-private partnerships are fostering collaborations to accelerate progress in cancer prevention,

treatment, and care. By working together, knowledge sharing and collective efforts can accelerate breakthroughs and advancements.

6. Prevention and Lifestyle Changes: A significant proportion of cancers are preventable through lifestyle modifications such as avoiding tobacco use, adopting healthy eating habits, engaging in regular physical activity, practicing sun protection, and receiving appropriate vaccinations. Promoting public awareness and implementing effective prevention strategies can significantly reduce cancer incidence rates.

7. Enhanced Supportive Care: Alongside advances in treatment,

there is increasing recognition of the importance of supportive care for cancer patients. Improved pain management, psychological support, palliative care, and survivorship programs contribute to enhancing the quality of life for individuals affected by cancer.

8. Rising Global Awareness: The growing awareness and understanding of cancer at both the individual and societal levels have led to increased support, funding, and advocacy for cancer research and initiatives. Governments, organizations, and communities are prioritizing cancer control and investing in programs aimed at

reducing the burden of cancer worldwide.

While the vision of a future without cancer remains ambitious, the progress achieved so far and the relentless efforts of the scientific and medical community give hope for continued advancements in prevention, detection, treatment, and support. By combining scientific knowledge, technological innovations, and collective determination, a future where cancer is less prevalent, more preventable, and better managed is within reach.

Epilogue: A Message Of Hope

In the journey through the pages of this book on cancer, we have explored the many facets of this complex disease. We have delved into its causes, risk factors, types, stages, and various treatment options. We have discussed the importance of early detection, lifestyle changes, and the incredible advancements in cancer research and treatment.

Amidst the vast array of information, one message shines through: hope. Hope is the unwavering belief that, together, we can conquer cancer. It is the fuel that drives researchers to unravel the mysteries of the disease, doctors to provide compassionate care, patients to persevere, and families to support one another.

In the face of cancer, hope is a beacon of light, guiding us through the darkest of times. It reminds us that there is strength in unity and solace in community. Hope lifts our spirits, encourages us to fight, and empowers us to embrace life with newfound appreciation.

We have witnessed the remarkable stories of cancer survivors who have defied the odds, their journeys becoming beacons of inspiration. These survivors teach us to never underestimate the power of the human spirit, the resilience that lies within each of us. They remind us that a cancer diagnosis does not define us but rather propels us to redefine what is possible.

Through the collective efforts of researchers, healthcare professionals, policymakers, and individuals, we have made incredible strides in the battle against cancer. New therapies, early detection methods, and prevention strategies continue to emerge, reshaping the landscape of cancer care.

In the future, we envision a world where cancer is a preventable and manageable condition. A world where every individual has access to effective treatments, compassionate care, and a support network to navigate the challenges. A world where the fear of cancer is replaced with hope, knowledge, and resilience.

But we cannot achieve this future alone. It requires a united front, where governments invest in cancer research, healthcare systems prioritize cancer care, and individuals take proactive steps to reduce their risk and support one another.

As we turn the final page of this book, let us carry the message of hope in our hearts. Let us stand together, unwavering in our commitment to prevent, detect, treat, and support those affected by cancer. Each of us has a role to play in the fight against cancer, whether as a survivor, caregiver, advocate, or supporter.

With hope as our guiding light, we embark on a future where the impact of cancer on individuals, families, and society is diminished. It may be a long and challenging journey, but together, we can create a world where the fear of cancer is replaced with hope, where lives are saved, and where the triumph of the human spirit shines bright.

Let us march forward with courage, resilience, and unwavering hope—a future without cancer awaits.

- Encouragement for those affected by cancer

To those who are facing the challenging road of cancer, or supporting a loved one on their journey, know that you are not alone. In the face of this disease, it is normal to feel overwhelmed, scared, and uncertain about what lies ahead.

But within you lies a wellspring of strength, resilience, and courage.

First and foremost, remember to be kind to yourself. Cancer can bring physical and emotional hardships, but it does not define who you are as a person. Allow yourself to feel a range of emotions, seek support from loved ones, and give yourself permission to rest and heal.

Surround yourself with a supportive network of family, friends, and healthcare professionals. They are there to provide a listening ear, lend a helping hand, and offer guidance throughout your journey. Lean on them, share your feelings, and let them lift you up when you need it most.

Stay informed, but be mindful of your individual needs. Educate yourself about your diagnosis and treatment options, but remember that every person's cancer journey is unique. Trust your medical team and engage in open and honest communication with them. They are your partners in this fight, and together, you can make informed decisions about your care.

Hold onto hope. Even in the darkest moments, hope can be a powerful force. It may come in different forms—whether it's the promise of new treatments, the support of loved ones, or the stories of other survivors who have triumphed over cancer. Allow hope to fuel your spirit, motivate you to keep going, and inspire you to find joy and meaning in each day.

Take care of yourself holistically. While medical treatments are essential, don't forget to address your physical, emotional, and spiritual well-being. Nurture your body with a balanced diet, regular exercise, and ample rest. Seek out counseling, support groups, or therapy to help navigate the emotional toll of cancer. Engage in activities that bring you joy, whether it's spending time in nature, pursuing hobbies, or practicing mindfulness.

Remember that you are more than your diagnosis. Cancer may be a part of your life, but it does not define your worth or limit your potential. Tap into your inner resilience, draw strength from the love and support around you, and believe in your ability to overcome this challenge.

Lastly, never lose sight of the progress being made in cancer research and treatment. Science is constantly advancing, and new breakthroughs are on the horizon. Medical advancements, innovative therapies, and improved support systems are continually transforming the landscape of cancer care.

You are not alone in this journey. There is a global community of individuals who have faced cancer, conquered it, and are standing with you. They are a testament to the power of the human spirit, the resilience of the body, and the hope that springs eternal.

You are stronger than you know, and you have the power to face this challenge head-on. Have faith in yourself, lean on your support system, and hold onto hope. You are capable of weathering this storm, and brighter days await you.

- Call to action for continued research and support

In the fight against cancer, we have made significant strides, but our work is far from over. The battle against this formidable disease requires ongoing research, support, and collective action. Here is a call to action for all of us:

1. Support Cancer Research: Advocate for increased funding for cancer research at both the government and private levels. Research is the cornerstone of progress in understanding cancer biology, developing new therapies, and improving patient outcomes. By supporting research institutions, organizations, and initiatives, we can drive breakthrough discoveries and accelerate the development of more effective treatments.

2. Promote Early Detection and Screening: Raise awareness about the importance of regular screenings for early cancer detection. Encourage

friends, family, and community members to undergo recommended screenings and follow-up appointments. Early detection significantly improves treatment outcomes and saves lives.

3. Foster Collaboration: Encourage collaboration among researchers, clinicians, and patients to share knowledge, data, and insights. Collaboration leads to a deeper understanding of cancer and accelerates the translation of research into clinical practice. By fostering an environment of collaboration, we can maximize the impact of our efforts and drive progress forward.

4. Advocate for Accessible and Affordable Cancer Care: Advocate

for policies that ensure equitable access to quality cancer care for all individuals, regardless of their socioeconomic status or geographic location. This includes affordable treatment options, comprehensive insurance coverage, and support services that address the physical, emotional, and financial needs of patients and their families.

5. Support Patient and Caregiver Well-being: Recognize the importance of supporting the well-being of cancer patients and their caregivers. This includes providing access to mental health resources, support groups, and survivorship programs. By prioritizing the holistic needs of patients and caregivers, we

can improve the overall quality of life during and after cancer treatment.

6. Raise Awareness and Reduce Stigma: Increase public awareness about cancer, its risk factors, and available resources. Education plays a vital role in empowering individuals to take proactive steps for prevention, early detection, and support. Additionally, work towards reducing the stigma associated with cancer, ensuring that those affected feel supported, understood, and embraced by their communities.

7. Promote Healthy Lifestyles: Encourage and promote healthy lifestyle choices that reduce the risk of cancer. This includes advocating for tobacco control measures,

promoting healthy eating habits, regular physical activity, sun protection, and other preventive measures. Small changes in our daily lives can have a significant impact on reducing cancer risk.

8. Support Cancer Organizations and Initiatives: Donate to reputable cancer organizations and initiatives that provide support services, advocacy, and research funding. These organizations play a vital role in advancing cancer care, supporting patients and families, and driving policy changes.

9. Share Stories and Inspire Others: Share your personal experiences or stories of resilience and survival to inspire others. Your journey may

offer hope, encouragement, and strength to those who are currently facing cancer. By sharing your story, you can make a difference in someone else's life.

10. Be an Advocate: Use your voice to advocate for policies, resources, and support systems that benefit cancer patients and their families. Write to your elected representatives, participate in awareness campaigns, and join advocacy groups to influence positive change in cancer care.

Remember, every action, no matter how small, contributes to the larger effort of fighting cancer. Together, we can make a difference. Let us unite, continue to support one

another, and work tirelessly towards
a future where cancer is no longer a
devastating force in our lives.

.....***.....

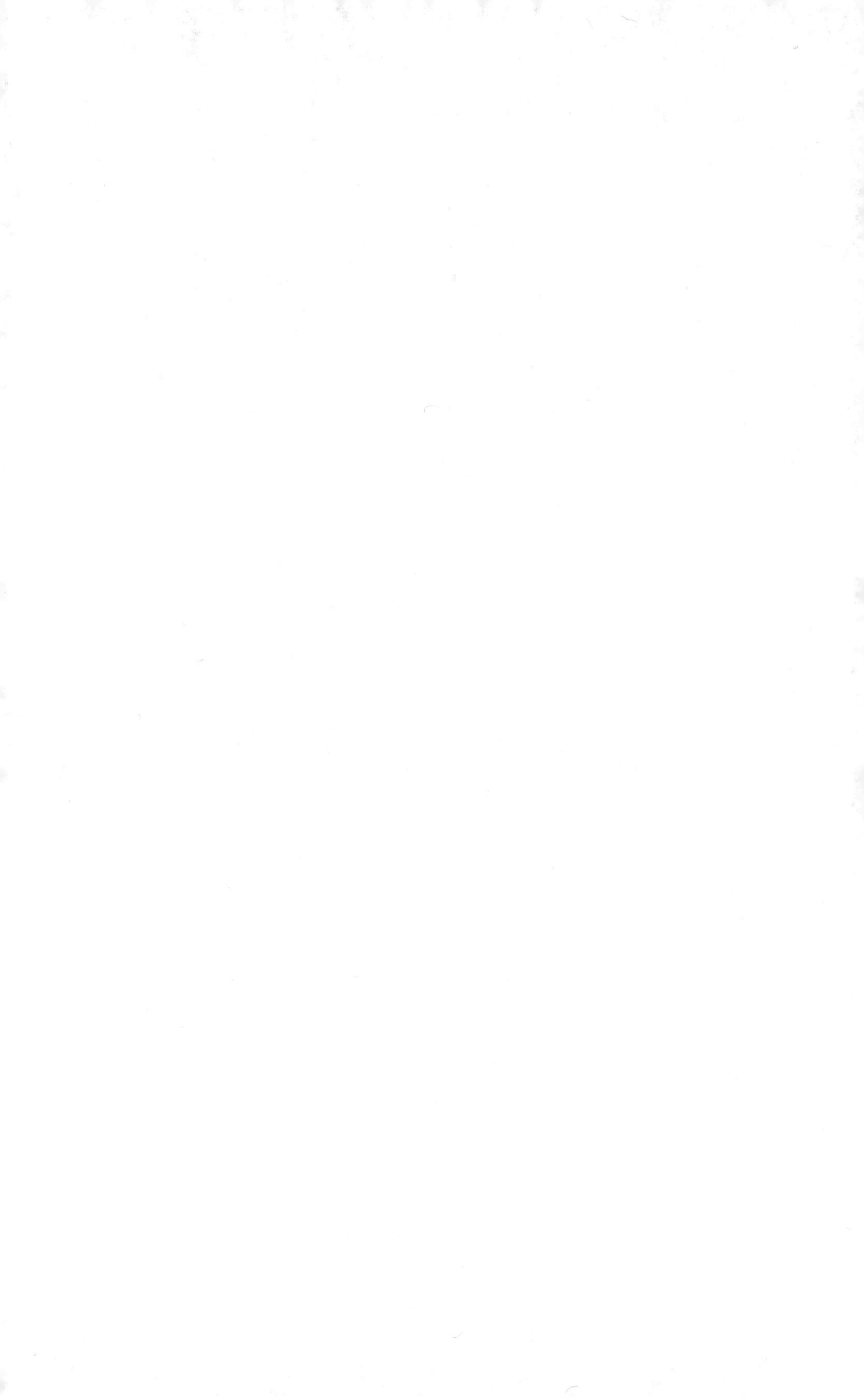